THE IMPLANT

Robert Ivey

Cover design by Robert Ivey

Dedication

This book is dedicated to all those who advocate
and fight for digital privacy rights.

CHAPTER ONE

Mel got her usual coffee — half regular and half decaf — from the barista and found her way to an empty table. Taking up a seat with her back to a wall and with a good view of the exits, she settled in to relax, people watch, catch up on the latest news, and perhaps come up with a story idea or two that would keep her freelance journalism going.

There was something about the atmosphere of the café that reminded her of comfort food. Maybe it was the aroma of recently baked pastries combined with coffee made from freshly ground beans and the whooshing sound coming from the espresso machine. Then again, it might be the seating areas with soft leather chairs and the murmurings of people in friendly conversation.

She hadn't been there five minutes when she noticed a man get up from a table across the room and appear to walk toward her. Seemingly in his mid-forties, he was clean-shaven and of average height and build. He wore jeans, a long-sleeved plaid shirt, and sneakers. A bit nerdy, she thought, whatever that means. Not thinking anything of it, she went back to studying her coffee, but was interrupted by the man standing by her table. He said, "Please excuse me, but aren't you Melinda Matthews?"

Looking up, she replied, "Yes, I am."

"Sorry to bother you, but could I have a word?" he asked.

Oh no, Mel thought, here it comes. The pickup line. And it's way too early in the day.

Sliding uninvited into the seat opposite Mel, he said, "I'm Dan Wilson and I think you are the only person I can talk to."

"Sorry, Mr. Wilson," Mel said. "You must have me confused with someone else. I'm sure there are other people who will listen to you. Besides, I'm not any kind of counselor."

"You're Melinda Matthews, the journalist, aren't you?"

"Yes, we've already been through that, so what do..."

"Then I have the right person," Dan interrupted. "I've read your work and feel that you are the only one I can confide in."

"There are priests and confessionals for that sort of thing."

"It's not that," Dan said. "I'm a scientist working for Gordon Pharmaceuticals. I've been working on the development of medical capsule implants. Perhaps you've heard of them."

5

"Yeah, I recall that they've been on the market for about a year now. Word has it that everyone is getting them."

"And soon we expect that they will become mandatory," Dan filled in, "but that is not what I wanted to talk to you about."

"Okay, you have my attention. Continue."

"You probably understand that they designed the capsule implant to monitor a person's health and send that data back to Gordon. Then Gordon's algorithms can combine that data with the person's DNA to develop personalized medication to treat an individual's medical problem. Sounds good, right?"

"I suppose. At least most people seem to buy into the idea without regard for the privacy implications."

"What most people don't know is that the capsules can track every person's location. And if that weren't bad enough, they can subtly deposit a message sent by Gordon and their government partners into a person's brain."

Mel was skeptical but played along. "So you're saying that these capsule implants can function as a mind-control device?"

"Exactly," Dan replied.

Thinking Dan was some crackpot, she asked, "Why are you telling me this and where is your proof?"

"I hoped that you would be as concerned as I am about our democracy and the direction our government is going and that you would report on this to warn the public."

"So I take it you want to come forward as a whistleblower?"

"I suppose so," Dan replied.

"You don't sound too sure."

"I've given this a lot of thought. Today when I saw you I thought it was time to act, but I have a family and am concerned for my life. These people are dangerous and determined."

"You're right to be concerned," Mel said, "but I can't publish a story on what you've just told me. I need proof and a lot of compelling, corroborating evidence."

Dan bent his head down toward the table. Looking up again, he said, "I understand. I will try to get you some proof."

Hoping that it wasn't a mistake, Mel handed Dan her business card and said, "Contact me when you have something."

Dan reciprocated and gave Mel his card, saying, "Thanks for listening to me." Then he got up and walked out.

Mel finished her now tepid coffee and made a few notes. She was hoping to get some story ideas when she came into the café, but what she just heard from Dan was unexpected. This was the story.

CHAPTER TWO

Several weeks passed. Mel had almost forgotten about her encounter with Dan Wilson but was reminded when she saw a message from him pop up in her email inbox. There were several attachments along with a brief message saying, "Here is the proof you are looking for, but if it gets out that I sent these, I'm a dead man."

Opening the attachments, Mel saw that they were design documents and letters with Gordon Pharmaceuticals' letterhead and logo.

So, good ole Dan must be legit after all, she thought.

Mel did a quick search of the U.S. Patent Office database. Sure enough, there they were in all their glorious legalese, describing an intelligent medical implant and monitoring system that included a communication device.

The name John Bender immediately came to mind as someone who could help her make sense of the patents and documents in the Dan email. Mel knew John from dorm parties while they were in college and had stayed in touch on a social level. Engineering and journalism seldom mixed, but John had a way of making complicated technical details seem simple, and that was just what Mel needed right now.

Mel sent John a text asking if they could meet and even offered to pay for lunch.

John replied, "Sure, when would be good? Always ready for a free lunch."

"How about tomorrow? Noon at Dave's? Free? You may have to work for this one."

"You're on," John replied. "See you there."

CHAPTER THREE

Mel waited for John outside Dave's Café and they went in together. After picking up their lunch orders — small salad and cup of soup for Mel, Cuban Panini for John — they made their way to a vacant table near the back.

As they settled in, they made some small talk — mostly it was John filling Mel in on his kids and family. All Mel had on her mind was her story and when John asked, "So what's up?" Mel was ready to lay it on him.

"First, have you gotten the medical capsule implant yet?" asked Mel.

"No, but I've been considering it," replied John.

"After you hear what I've learned, you may want to reconsider." Then Mel told John, in a hushed voice, about the meeting with Dan without revealing his full name, company, the documents he sent, or her patent search.

"So how can I help?" John asked.

"I would like you to look over the documents I got from Dan," Mel said, "and give me your best evaluation of what you think the social implications are given the technology involved. Is Dan right to be concerned?"

Handing John a sticky note with the relevant patent numbers written on it, Mel said, "I thought this was the best way for you to get started. Please get back to me when you have something."

CHAPTER FOUR

Mel received a text message from John two weeks after their meeting, saying that he had some information for her.

Letting John into her apartment, Mel said, "Thanks for coming over."

Settling into her work space in the bay window area of her living room overlooking the street, she showed John the documents Dan provided on her computer. "I didn't want to show you these at Dave's the other day because public Wi-Fi is notoriously insecure."

"I understand," John replied. "Give me some time to look over these."

Mel retreated to the kitchen to make some tea and prepare something for lunch, but she could not be still and paced the floor feeling the jitters of anxiety.

"Could you please settle down?" John asked.

"Sorry," Mel said. "But this is a big scoop for me. One that could bump my career up a notch or two or maybe lead to a Pulitzer."

About an hour had passed before John said, "Okay, let's talk about what I've learned from going over these documents and patents."

"First, this is a pretty sophisticated and potentially dangerous device. You're right to be concerned. At the heart of the device is a group of sensors that provide a full range of bodily monitoring much like you would get from a typical blood lipid profile at a commercial lab along with other measurements like heart rate."

"But haven't such devices been around for a while?" asked Mel.

"Yes," John replied. "Over the years there have been many implantable chips, meds with built-in sensors to notify the doctor when the patient had taken their prescribed medication. These include pacemakers and even wearable devices that monitor various bodily functions. Most notably, these devices send their data using short-range Bluetooth technology to your smartphone, which then forwards that data on to your doctor over the internet. What's new with the capsule is the range of the measurements being taken and that the capsules can communicate directly through the internet over the medical implant communications service band without having to relay their data through a smartphone. This technology provides a system and method for the implant to communicate directly with a medical controller, in this case Gordon's computers."

"But isn't the capability to have a person's bodily data constantly available to the medical professionals without going to the trouble of getting periodic lab tests something that people want?" Mel asked.

"I suppose so," John said. "To me, what makes this troubling is that now everyone with one of these implanted capsules will be directly addressable over the internet. In other words, each person will now be assigned their own unique internet address."

"We seem to have reached the ultimate in the era of the 'internet of things'," Mel said, "where people have become just another thing on the internet; for people who are online 24/7, their entire lives will become just another commodity available for exploitation at will by any business or government."

"Another thing that's new," John continued, "and I must emphasize, something that's very innovative, is how the capsule is powered. It's using body chemistry to serve as a battery. That's unlike the previous technology that had built-in power sources with a short life or used external batteries or an implantable radio frequency ID-like device that relied on induced power from the outside like those pads you lay your smartphone on to charge them. As long as you are alive, the body is powering the capsule.

These capsules also have a built-in location tracker. Think about it, constant connection to the internet and the ability to track your location 24/7. Chipped like an animal being monitored in the wild."

"But this is not new," Mel said. "The ability to track a person's location is available in every computing device we have like our smartphones, laptops, and e-readers. It is this capability that businesses exploit to send you ads when you pass by their stores and makes it easier for the government to find you."

"I agree," replied John. "The difference with the implant, though, is that people cannot turn it off, not that many disable tracking even with the existing technology. There will no longer be any place where a person can hide or even be alone unless you're willing to lock yourself up in an electromagnetically shielded room. That doesn't sound like much of a life to me."

"Sounds like George Orwell's *1984*," Mel remarked.

"The worst is yet to come. Are you ready for this?"

"Lay it on me," Mel said.

"The last function of the implant capsule and the subject of one of its patents is its use as a mind-control device. Basically, several electrodes on the device stimulate the nerves in the brain stem where the device is implanted to either induce headache-like pain or convey a message. To most people, this message would be almost indistinguishable from those little voices called inner speech that we all hear when we're thinking or silently reading. Some people prefer to claim that this inner speech is their God talking to them. Imagine how powerful this will be in the hands of government."

"Wow," Mel said. "I guess whistleblower Dan was right. We must do something. The public has to be warned. What do you think we should do?"

"I don't know. I'm just a poor engineer. You're the one with the contacts to reach the public. One thing I know, I'm sure not going to get the implant."

"Good, I thought you would feel that way," Mel said.

They both sat silently for a while, immersed in their own thoughts about the next actions and their consequences.

"Are you going to publish a story about this?"

"I can't just yet. Most publications these days want some kind of personal angle, so I need to do some interviews with people who have the implant."

CHAPTER FIVE

Mel remembered that when she met some friends at lunch a month ago, Alison discussed experiencing some strange sensations after getting an implant. Everyone was sympathetic but thought no more of it. Now Mel wanted to learn more.

After the exchange of a few text messages, they agreed to meet for dinner at The White Rhino in Shadyside on Friday evening. By the time they arrived, the only table available was a high-top in the bar area. Mel chose the stool facing the bar, so she could see anyone approaching her from behind in the bar mirror. With the clamor of patrons and the ever-present TV screens tuned to different sports channels, the place was noisy, but that was fine with Mel —less chance for people to eavesdrop on their conversation.

"So how have you been?" Mel asked Alison.

"Busy and hectic as usual, what with the kids and work," Alison replied. "So glad you got in touch. It's been a while and I sure needed a break."

"The last time we met you mentioned some strange sensations after receiving your implant. Is that still a problem?"

"Well, I've sort of gotten used to it. It's just part of the 'new normal', so they say, even though I hate that phrase. How about you?"

"I'm working on a big story about the implants and thought of what you told us when we last got together with Becky and Tasha. Please forgive me, I don't mean to pry, but I was wondering if you would be willing to share your experience?"

"Off the record?" Alison asked.

"Of course," Mel replied. She assured Alison that if she was uncomfortable, they could just forget it and have a leisurely dinner talking about something else.

"No, that's okay. I've been wanting to talk to someone about what I've experienced," Alison said. "Now please don't think I've gone all schizoid and paranoid, but I've had the feeling that I'm being watched all the time... and I keep hearing voices in my head."

"But we all have that inner voice going on in our heads. For some of us it is hard to turn it off and get some relief," Mel offered somewhat jokingly.

"Yes, but since getting the implant, my inner voice, if you want to call it that, is different. For example, in the last election, the voice kept telling me to vote for that idiot Frank Unger, something I would never have thought pre-implant. After the election, that message was gone. Very strange, I thought."

"What's the voice telling you these days?"

"Besides the incessant and annoying ads, the voice is strongly and repeatedly telling me to go to rallies to support one politician or another and to support issues I'm not in favor of. Mel, I'm a working mother with two kids and a husband. It's all we can do to pay the bills, keep a roof over our heads and food on the table. I don't have time for the foolishness the voice is asking of me. I've heard from others that some people now claim that the voice they are hearing is the voice of God. Others have gone so far as to make it into a religion, fools that they are."

"Welcome to the era of so-called surveillance capitalism and surveillance politics," Mel said with a touch of sarcasm.

Alison gave Mel a crooked grin as Mel asked, "Have you considered having the implant removed?"

"Yes, I've heard that there are doctors who will do that, but the reason I agreed to the implant was because my insurance company said that they would drop me if I didn't go through with the procedure... and I can't afford to be without the insurance."

"Sorry, I didn't mean to get you upset. You have been very helpful, so how about we just chill and enjoy our drinks and dinner? So, what are your kids up to?"

CHAPTER SIX

After John's analysis of the documents
provided by Dan and the revelations offered by her
friend Alison, Mel was more determined than ever
to expose the medical monitor capsule implant for
what it truly was — a privacy-invading mind-
control device.

Remembering a story she had done earlier
on hacktivism, Mel contacted Damon. Maybe he
could develop a way to hack into Gordon's
computer network to stop the tracking and mind-
control messages.

Mel: *Hi Damon, U remember me?*

Damon: *Yes, How could I forget? ur story
got me into a lot of trouble.*

Mel: *Sorry, really need ur help. Can we meet?*

Damon: *K come on over.*

Mel made her way to Damon's third-floor walk-up apartment and knocked on the door.

Damon let her into a room of threadbare furniture and a few cheap throw rugs. Most of the flat surfaces were covered with empty glasses, cans from a wide variety of soft drink and beer companies, paper plates, and takeout containers.

Damon's apartment decor matched his unkempt appearance, which included a long beard that looked to hold the remains of several past meals.

Dominating one side of the room was a floor to ceiling pile of both ancient and modern computers in states that varied from just a collection of parts to active screens flashing what appeared to be a scroll of incomprehensible text and messages. This teetering monument to Damon's passion was obviously his pride and joy.

"Thanks for seeing me," Mel said. "Before we get started, I need to know if they have implanted you."

"No." Knowing full well what Mel, meant he added jokingly, "Just a couple of teeth." He then asked, "Have you?"

"No," Mel said.

Mel gave Damon the executive summary of what she found out about the capsule implant device, being careful not to reveal any of her sources.

"These devices are dangerous. Gordon and the government need to be stopped for the good of our country and our way of life. Would you be interested in hacking into the implant messaging system at Gordon to stop the mind-control messages and the tracking?"

"I can try to gain access to Gordon's systems and deposit a virus that will stop the messages for a time, but don't underestimate Gordon or the government. They have very smart people and a lot more resources than me. So, what I do will only be, to them, a temporary glitch. Inevitably, they will find the virus and then block and remove it. Worse, they may track me down and eliminate me."

Trying to appeal to Damon's sense of patriotism, Mel said, "So, for the sake of our country are you willing to at least try it?"

"Okay, sounds like a challenge, and you know how I like a challenge. I'll see what I can do, but what are you doing? Seems like we should alert the people. This problem needs to be attacked from both directions. Right?"

"You're correct," Mel said. "I have written an article describing the dangerous implications of the implant and hope to get it published soon. Maybe it will arouse the public to take action."

"Good luck with that. The public are sheep and have fallen prey to the propaganda touting the medical benefits of the device. And with health care costs what they are along with their suffering at the hands of pharmaceuticals that cause more harm than good, they are desperately grasping at solutions. The revelations in your article will probably not dissuade them much."

"Well, we have to try."

CHAPTER SEVEN

Mel worked all night on her medical monitor capsule implant story. She submitted it at 6:00 AM via email to Ben Rosen, the editor at the *Times Herald,* along with the info to verify her confidential sources. Mel had submitted many other stories to her hometown newspaper and found Ben to be tough but supportive and always on the lookout for interesting and news breaking stories. She was hopeful and confident that this story would lead as a breaking news story and not just another filler or opinion piece.

With thoughts of a Pulitzer running through her mind, Mel settled on her couch with a cup of coffee, too wound up to get any sleep. Perhaps coffee was not the right choice of drink given she was already feeling jittery with anticipation and it was still early morning.

She didn't have to wait long before she received a text message from Ben requesting she come into the office for a meeting. Mel replied that she was on her way.

* * *

Arriving at Ben's office at 9:00 AM she gave a courtesy knock on his office door. He motioned for her to come in saying, "Close the door and have a seat."

Ben looked at Mel over his glasses from across his desk and said, "Your piece is very good but..."

Here it comes, Mel thought. What could possibly be wrong? Why the "but?" She knew Ben to be fair in providing constructive criticism. That was it, she was sure of it.

Ben continued while Mel's mind wandered. "We can't publish it."

"What?" Mel said. "Why not?"

"You may not be aware, but this publication is owned by Alex Gordon through several Caribbean shell companies. If we publish your exposé, Gordon will shut us down."

Mel's jaw nearly hit the floor, but she recovered enough to say, "I didn't mention Gordon in my article or make any accusations."

"No, you didn't have to, but you exposed the dangers of the capsule and everyone knows that Gordon has a monopoly on the device, so you may as well have."

So much for freedom of the press, Mel thought.

"Then I will just have to publish the piece elsewhere," Mel said.

"As a freelancer, you are, of course, free to do that," Ben replied. "But just between you and me, please be careful. People like Gordon and his henchman are dangerous and his being in bed with our corrupt government can complicate your situation. Watch your back."

On her way home, the growling in her stomach reminded Mel that she had had no breakfast and she was starving. Stopping at Dave's Café for a bite to eat and more coffee, she reflected on what Ben had said about watching your back. That was something she always did following the lessons learned as a young girl from her late father, a career CIA agent.

So, what now? Mel thought. Taking out her pen and tablet, she jotted down a few notes. Among these was a list of some publications she had previously submitted articles to. Suddenly she had an epiphany. Why not use social media and perhaps a website to get the message out? It was so obvious. Why didn't I think of it before?

* * *

Arriving back at her apartment, Mel immediately got to work and sent her article to three publications that accepted freelance work. Then she set up a social media site using the ID @BanTheCap being careful to protect her privacy by not filling out the personal details on the sign-up screen and opting out of all ads.

CHAPTER EIGHT

Mel's smartphone pinged, announcing a new message. It was Damon.

Damon: *Did the hack. u ready to talk?*

Mel: *K, where/when?*

Damon: *9am tomorrow at Dave's.*

Mel: *K, c u there.*

The next day Mel went to Dave's. After getting her coffee she slid into the chair opposite Damon who was hunkered down behind his laptop.

"So, what do you have?" Mel asked.

"See the tall guy in slacks and a blue shirt who just came in?" Damon asked.

"Yes. What about him?"

"I'll bet he orders a mocha latte."

"How do you know?"

"I've been coming here for two weeks now and take up a spot where I can see what people order." Tapping a box about the size of a deck of cards, he said, "Every day I set my laptop up with a Wi-Fi router known as a man-in-the-middle-attack. When people with the implant come in, their internet address will appear on my computer. It will then communicate through my router, so I can capture everything the implant sends and receives. The internet-of-things devices like these implants have no effective security or firewalls."

Mel listened intently as Damon continued.

"Since I can communicate with their implant, I can alter the medical data it sends back to Gordon or I can send it a message telling them what to order. It works most of the time, but some people are just stubborn and ignore the message." Damon turned the laptop so Mel could see the screen and pointed at a line of numbers in what looked like a spreadsheet. "See, this is our guy."

"How do you know that the people have ordered what you told them to... and that it is not just their favorite?"

"A lot of the people who come in here are regulars, and I make a note of what they order. Then one day I will send a message for them to order something different, and like I said, most of them do. I know that it's not all that scientific."

"I'm impressed," said Mel.

"But that's not all," Damon continued. "I've developed a logic bomb that I have sent to Gordon through the medical implant service channel masquerading as a packet of medical data. It will go off in a week and we will see what happens."

"Great job," said Mel. "I owe you big time, thanks."

CHAPTER NINE

"10 Million Medical Records Hacked" read the headline. The story read like a press release from Gordon Pharmaceuticals, saying that patient records in their database had been compromised and would prevent them from providing their custom-made medication to their customers. The article made a big point to condemn the perpetrator and promised swift apprehension and prosecution equating the attack as an act of terrorism.

As Mel read this story, she knew that Damon's logic bomb had gone off as planned.

The article explained that hackers had deleted or changed some medical records. This would delay plans to make the implant mandatory for all citizens until the vulnerabilities in the system had been corrected. It would also delay further delivery of custom medications. This would adversely affect the health and very survival of many implant subscribers.

Customers? Subscribers? Mel thought. These are just capitalistic euphemisms that referred to an insidious movement toward mass surveillance.

Mel felt bad about the health implications, but she thought it would take an event like this to wake people up to the growing threat of the surveillance state and then rebel against it.

People were up in arms, so to speak, and were scrambling to find alternative needed medications. Even though it only took a few days for Gordon's people to restore his systems from backups, he spun this event to further strengthen the need for and the criticality of the medical implant capsules in the minds of the public.

CHAPTER TEN

The text message on Mel's phone from Damon read: *see me ASAP*.

When Mel reached Damon's third-floor walk-up apartment, she found the door ajar. Pushing the door open slowly, she looked in and listened for any intruders. Feeling it was safe, she made her way inside. The place was a shambles, noticeably more so than Damon's normal living conditions. She saw tossed furniture, a flipped mattress, dresser drawers dumped, the contents of kitchen cabinets and the refrigerator swept out onto the floor, and holes punched into the walls. Whoever did this was looking for something, just being destructive, or both. Among the debris, Mel saw Damon's pile of destroyed computers. Though it was hard to tell, she thought some of his equipment was missing. But where was Damon?

Mel texted Damon: *I'm at ur apt where r u?*

The reply came quickly. Damon: *At the airport. Meet me at café in front of security.*

It was a 40-minute ride to the airport, but Mel found Damon nursing a latte at the café.

"I was worried about you. What's going on? Your apartment was severely trashed and some of your equipment seemed to be missing."

"I told you I feared for my life after hacking into Gordon's systems. A few days ago I noticed that I was being followed. This morning when I looked down on the street, I saw two black SUV vehicles pull up in front of the building and some very tough looking dudes came in. They didn't look like any residents or visitors I'd ever seen. That meant only one thing. They were coming for me. So, I grabbed my bug-out-bag, went out the back way, jumped the fence and made it here."

"So, what are you going to do now?" Mel asked.

Giving a nod over to the nearby TSA check-point, Damon said, "I'm planning to leave the country and visit with friends in Europe. If I'm lucky, Gordon and his government cronies will not have issued an alert and their facial recognition systems will not flag me."

"Those are big ifs," Mel said. "Are you going to be okay?"

"I know you couldn't afford to pay me, but I made out big time by selling the vulnerabilities I found in Gordon's systems and the capsules."

"Vulnerabilities?" Mel asked.

"Yeah, think of a vulnerability as a hole or flaw in a system's software that can be filled by someone like me to access data in other parts of a system or cause damage in the form of a virus or malware. These vulnerabilities are like gold in the marketplace for such things. I expect that Gordon will be fighting off hackers for some time."

"I'd like to stay and chat, but I have a plane to catch," Damon added.

As Damon got up to leave, Mel said, "Thanks for your help and good luck."

Mel watched as Damon joined the crush of travelers in the intestine-shaped maze leading into the security check-point.

CHAPTER ELEVEN

The social media campaign for Ban-The-Cap had been active for three weeks. And it surprised Mel how well it was going thanks in part to a blog post she made of the same article that Ben Rosen at the *Times Herald* had rejected. Shortly after it was picked up by an online newsfeed website.

The hundreds of comments that were pouring in daily from across the country of implanted people encouraged Mel. Many of them told their stories of mysterious feelings of being watched and of strange internal thoughts — thoughts not only of what political positions to take but of what products to buy. But even the non-implantees voiced serious concerns and accused Gordon and the government of colluding to implement a "Big Brother" society where individual privacy had ceased to exist.

Even though people suffered from what they perceived as the "side effects" of the implant, they defended the medical monitoring aspects of the device saying that the resulting custom medications had improved their lives.

Incentivized by a deal that Gordon made with the government to reduce a person's medical insurance if they agreed to be implanted, people were clamoring to get it. So much so that most medical facilities performing the procedure were overwhelmed.

As a writer, Mel had preferred to stay in the background, creating articles of interest and doing copy-writing work which brought in the bulk of her modest income. She never thought of herself as an activist and never wanted to take on that role.

Yet here she was in a position of trying to organize people and lead protests against what she saw as a big business and government conspiracy to destroy democracy and in effect reduce the entire population into a mass of compliant followers serving an authoritarian oligarchy.

Before Damon left the country, Mel had worked with him to set up a website called The Digital Privacy Network. This website made use of a secure organizing tool specifically designed for activists. This made it easier for Mel to communicate with others around the country and to announce protest events. The website along with the sister BanTheCap social media platform grew to 50,000 followers from across the country almost overnight. It was time for action, which meant taking the message to the streets and to the elected representatives.

While the social media websites showed success in getting the word out, they were not without the downside posed by trolls and threats. Every day Mel saw comments threatening to kill her, kidnap her, or hurt her family. Some even so vile as to say, "I am gonna rape you to death." Many of these she reported to the police, but they were powerless to find and prosecute the perpetrators, mostly because these messages came from fake accounts generated by bots and trolls. The trolls, however, covered their tracks well.

* * *

Mel and her friend Tasha organized the first protest rally, which they had scheduled to take place in front of the Gordon Pharmaceuticals headquarters on Second Avenue.

When they arrived, there were already about 100 people milling about all dressed in various forms of "Stealth Wear" to conceal themselves from surveillance. Most were holding homemade signs with the now familiar BanTheCap logo and slogans saying: "Return our Privacy," "Digital Freedom," and "Digital Privacy Now."

On the opposite side of the street were an equal number of people brandishing signs saying "Keep the Cap" and "Health care is our right." Some were shouting slogans and threats against Mel's protesters.

"Do you think Alex is in there and watching?" Tasha asked.

"I expect so," said Mel. "His private helicopter is parked on the roof and the building is just bristling with closed-circuit TV cameras."

The city had permitted the peaceful demonstration for two hours in the morning. Gordon was prepared with police and company security dressed out in full riot gear ready to meet the protesters. The media was also present and being a media person herself Mel took advantage of the several stand up interviews to get the word out about the truth behind the implant capsules.

Mel was encouraging the protesters through a bullhorn when someone grabbed her shoulder from behind and forcefully turned her around. Facing the person, she was surprised to see that it was her estranged brother holding a "Keep The Cap" sign. "Jason, what are you doing here?" Mel asked as she brushed his hand away.

Jason replied, "I could ask you the same thing. Why are you trying to deprive people of their right to health care?"

"We are not protesting to deprive anyone of their health care. We just don't think compromising and monetizing people's personal data should be part of the picture," Mel said. "We'll to continue protesting until your boss changes the capsules to remove the tracking and mind-control features and stops invading people's privacy."

Screaming over the noise of the protesters on both sides, Jason said, "My boss? You think Alex Gordon is my boss? I'm here counter-protesting in favor of this new technology that will provide people with much needed advanced health care, including myself."

Mel yelled back. "We can't talk here. You know where I live."

Mel and Jason had been estranged since they were teens when Mel shared a confidence with him and he had used it against her. Mel had never forgotten the incident and could not bring herself to forgive him. He had betrayed a trust and that was unforgivable.

Mel had just turned around to face her group when suddenly Alex's mob of counter-protesters surged forward, forcefully engaging her group. What had started as a peaceful protest turned into an all-out scuffle with the police intervening to restore order.

After being knocked down and kicked repeatedly during the melee, Mel crawled across the street to the curb and found some safety against a black stone wall.

Mel looked up to see a bloody Tasha fleeing for safety and shouted, "Tasha, please help me."

"Mel, is that you?" she asked. "You look terrible. Sorry I didn't see you."

"Let's get you some medical attention," Tasha said as she helped Mel to her feet.

There were no EMTs on-site, so they limped to Mel's car in a parking garage a couple blocks away. They drove to the nearest hospital a short distance across the river where Mel and Tasha were patched up in the ER and then released.

CHAPTER TWELVE

Tasha helped Mel into her apartment and eased her onto the couch.

Mel ached from the bruising to her abdomen and rib cage, not to mention the lacerations to her head that ER staff stitched up along with many scrapes and small cuts. It relieved her to know she didn't have any broken bones.

"Can I get you anything?" Tasha asked.

Mel said, "There's some wine in the fridge. I know it's early, but maybe you could pour us both a glass and then we can lick our wounds over today's disaster."

Tasha set the two glasses of wine on the coffee table. As she took a seat in a chair opposite

Mel, she asked, "Who was that guy you were talking to."

"That was my brother, Jason."

"I didn't know that you had a brother," Tasha said.

"We've been estranged since we were teens, and I haven't seen or heard from him in years. It's a long story."

"So, what went wrong today?" Tasha asked.

"I was not prepared for an organized opposition," Mel said. "I should have seen it coming because the social media threads for several weeks now have been growing with opposing views from people following the Keep-the-Cap hashtag group, not to mention many outright hate messages and threats."

"Do you think Alex Gordon is at the root of this opposition effort?"

"I have no doubt. As we were protesting, I could almost envision him looking out over the near-riot and gloating."

"Okay, so what went right?"

"I was encouraged that so many like-minded people showed up, though we should have had more signs and t-shirts to give out. Also, I hope that Alex now realizes that he has a fight on his hands."

"What's next?"

"Well, we have another demonstration in two weeks in front of the Federal Building if our permit is not withdrawn. I have no idea if today's fiasco will result in larger or smaller numbers, but we are going ahead with it permit or not."

"But right now, I really need to get some rest. The meds they gave me in the ER and the wine are having their effect. After that, I will write up my first-person account of the demonstration.

Maybe Rosen at the *Times* will publish it. If not, a blog post will have to do for now."

Tasha left, and Mel faded off to sleep on the couch. Waking in a daze some twelve hours later, Mel looked out on the now dark street and set to work composing a report documenting her first-person account of the happenings at the demonstration. Maybe I can get it finished in time to submit it to Rosen in the morning, she thought.

CHAPTER THIRTEEN

Jason was hesitant about visiting Mel and had walked back and forth in front of her apartment for 15 agonizing minutes, trying to get up the nerve to knock on her door. The last time Jason and Mel had seen each other, besides the demonstration, was at their mother's funeral. Of course, the tension of either event was not conducive to any kind of reconciliation.

Mel opened her door and the two of them stared expressionless at each other for what seemed like forever. Finally, she motioned for him to come in without so much as one kind word of welcome.

"Are you all right?" Jason asked.

"A bit banged up, but I'm on the mend," Mel replied.

"Sorry about the scuffle. I don't know how it got started."

"Scuffle?" Mel asked. "It was all out-war and it was totally uncalled for."

"You're right," Jason said. "Somehow passions got out of control but that is not an excuse."

"Do you have the implant?" Mel asked.

"Yes," replied Jason. "You?"

"No," Mel said. "Why do you have the implant?"

"I've contracted an incurable blood condition. The custom-tailored medication from Gordon has restored my ability to live a normal life with my symptoms under control and without the debilitating side effects caused by the traditional medications. Many of the protesters on my side are in a similar situation, so I hope you can see how they might have gotten overzealous."

"Overzealous?" Mel shot back. "People were injured in what was intended to be a peaceful protest. There's no excuse for that kind of behavior."

Mel sat in silence for a moment to cool off, then after taking some deep breaths asked, "Aren't you at all bothered about giving up your privacy to a company and then having them exploit your every private action to serve their advertising and political agenda?"

"Yes, that's the annoying part. But most people I know with the implant have learned to ignore it or are in denial or just consider it a small price to pay in exchange for their medical treatment."

"It seems strangely coincidental that you were at the demonstration," said Mel.

Jason gave Mel that sheepish look that she recognized from their childhood, --that look of guilt, as if he had done something wrong. "Why do you say that?" asked Jason.

"Are you working for Alex Gordon?"

"N...n...n-o," Jason lied. Well, it was only a partial lie. He had never met or talked to Alex in person, but he had been contacted by Alex's associates who wanted him to spy and report back on Mel's activities. At first, he refused, but he needed the money. With the amount they offered, he could pay off his bills along with his ballooning credit card debt and still have some left so he could start over somewhere.

"So why do you want to destroy the advances that have been made with the capsule and personalized medication technology?" Jason asked.

"I don't want to lessen the benefits that this technology has delivered to those who need it, but like I said before, I believe that personal privacy is a right and should be honored and treated as sacrosanct."

Both Mel and Jason realized that this discussion was going nowhere, so Jason said, "I think your position has been influenced by what happened when we were teens. I think you are still pissed at me for betraying your trust."

"You're damn right I'm pissed at you. You came here not because of any concern for my wellbeing or to try to patch things up between us. You came here trying to get information on my plans so you can provide feedback to Alex. You came here to spy on me. You came here to betray my trust again. Right? I think it's time you left."

Jason said nothing. He just walked out with his head down.

CHAPTER FOURTEEN

While it was difficult to keep up with the social media comments after the first protest rally, the media exposure emboldened Mel to forge ahead.

During the weeks leading up to the next local demonstration at the Federal Building where several local politicians had their offices, the number of social media followers grew to 100,000. Mel and her team had scheduled demonstrations in a dozen other cities, including Washington D.C. During this time, the donations coming into the crowd-source website grew to $60,000. This was enough to supply other demonstration groups with placards and t-shirts.

Bolstered by news articles in the press along with the websites and social media feeds, Mel found herself in a position of power that she didn't seek. She developed a following because she had identified for the people a common enemy and provided forums to fight that enemy. In this new role as leader of this movement, she, along with a team of volunteer leaders in other cities, took on the huge task of organizing the protests by providing the logistics and letting followers know where and when to show up for a protest rally.

The largest rally to date was held on the National Mall in Washington D.C. a short 6 months after the first rally with some 150,000 protesters taking part. This event included a makeshift stage provided by volunteers with a schedule of speakers and musical entertainment. While the rally was going on, Mel and a team of volunteers combed the halls of legislative power targeting Senators and Congressman, hoping for a few minutes to communicate their message about the intrusive nature of the medical implant capsules. But like the many messages the representatives had previously received through massive email and letter writing-campaigns, the elected officials were as unmoved and dismissive as always. When it came to responding to the voice of the people, the representatives preferred instead to favor those voices from lobbying groups and big business.

CHAPTER FIFTEEN

Mel felt fortunate to live in a community where many small shops were within easy walking distance from her apartment. Most every day she went to her favorite coffee shop for her morning eye-opener, but today this was not to be.

She was within a block of the shop when she noticed two well-dressed but muscular-looking men in dark suits following close behind her. She picked up her pace, but it was no use. The thugs stayed close on her tail.

In the middle of the block, she saw what appeared to be a delivery van with its side door open. As she passed by, the two thugs grabbed hold of her and hustled her into the van. It happened so fast that she didn't have time to scream for help before they gagged her.

The short ride across town ended at a back loading dock entrance to Gordon Pharmaceuticals.

* * *

The door to Alex Gordon's expansive office opened and the two thugs frog-marched Mel in. Freeing her from their grip, she stood there while the thugs took up their posts next to the door.

To say that Alex's corner office was expansive would be an understatement since the square footage was at least as much as that of two average-sized homes.

At one end was a large glass-topped desk with no drawers and void of anything except a lamp and a walnut and gold pen set. At the other was a conference table surrounded by perhaps ten chairs. In between were several settings of couches and chairs arranged on ornate Asian-designed carpets, the only color in an otherwise sterile office space.

Rising from his plush, high-backed chair behind his desk, Alex walked over to Mel. Extending his hand, he said in a condescending tone, "Welcome, little lady."

Mel felt her face flush. Refusing to take his proffered hand, she told him in a forceful tone of voice, "First, I'm not your little lady. And what's the meaning of having your thugs kidnap me off the street?"

Unfazed, Alex said, "Come in and have a seat." He gestured to the chairs in front of his desk.

Mel saw that the guest chairs were noticeably lower than Alex's desk chair. Refusing to be put into a subordinate position, she said, "No thanks, I'll stand."

"You must be thirsty after your ordeal at the hands of my associates. I know that they can be a bit rough at times. Would you like something to drink?"

"No," Mel replied. "I demand that you release me immediately."

Walking over to a built-in glass and stainless-steel credenza, Alex poured himself a glass of water from a crystal pitcher on a silver tray.

Alex turned to Mel with a wide, toothy smile and said, "You are in no position to be making demands. You have been causing me a lot of trouble, and you are here for us to have a frank discussion about that. You should keep in mind that I could've just as easily had you eliminated, but I'm a reasonable man and thought we should have a talk first."

Walking along what appeared to be a blank wall, Alex waved his hand. The wall opened up, as if by magic, to reveal an elevator.

"Let me give you a tour of our facility," Alex said. "We can walk and talk."

Mel did not have much choice since the two thugs were right behind her ushering her into the elevator.

Four floors below Alex's office, the doors opened onto a long passageway with windows lining both sides. As soon as Alex stepped into the walkway, the lights on the factory floor below came on automatically.

Gesturing to his left, Alex said, "This is where we make the implant capsules and on the other side is where we manufacture the personalized medicines."

What struck Mel about the entire facility was that there were no humans in sight; machines and robots ran the entire operation. While this was not that unusual in this age of total automation, it was the scale of the facility that was breathtaking.

With some obvious pride, Alex said, "What you are looking at is the only manufacturing facility making these products in the world. I don't understand why you and your followers are so set on destroying all of this."

Attempting to appeal to Alex's ego, Mel replied, "What you have built here including the design and use of the implant capsule are impressive, but you must realize that your ingenious device represents a huge invasion of privacy and a violation of an individual's natural and constitutional rights."

"Beginning in the era of social media, the masses willingly gave up their privacy," Alex said. "The people have been easily led down the path toward accumulating friends and followers, virtual or not. In exchange for their privacy, they became the focus of marketers who appealed to their insatiable accumulation desires along with luring them into like-minded political and cultural silos of thought. We are just capitalizing on the public's follower mentality to use their personal information to improve their lives and our civilization. And, by the way, we are aware of your ban-the-cap social media campaign to organize people against us."

"Improve their lives?" Mel replied. "As altruistic as your words sound, what you and your fellow oligarchs really want is a compliant public who will do your bidding including the buying of the products and ideas that you and your buddies are luring them into."

"Oligarchs? We have been fortunate to gather the resources necessary to improve the lives of millions. So why not do it? So what if we make a buck or two in the process?"

"But at what cost?" asked Mel.

"Everything has a cost," Alex said. "And in this case the cost is privacy."

"That is unacceptable, and we will fight you and your kind every step of the way."

As soon as she said it, Mel realized she may have spoken in haste and overplayed her hand.

Alex almost spit as he shot back. "With what, little lady? You have no power or resources."

As they continued down the glass-enclosed passageway, Alex pointed out the computer center with its banks of cabinets, each with a multitude of tiny blinking lights.

"This is just one of four computer centers we have built in the country to track people and design the personalized medicines that some of them need to survive. These centers rival the size and scope of those used by the National Security Administration and those run by the companies providing cloud services."

Alex continued, "With the fast pace of technological advancement, people are rapidly becoming useless because of their lack of skills or their inability to continue to learn new skills as technology evolves. The result is a growing class of people who have become economically irrelevant. So, what's a government to do to manage all these useless people and prevent social unrest? Like a toddler who needs parents to take care of them and look out for their needs, the implant we have developed communicates directly with our computers so it can learn each person's likes and dislikes. Then it feeds them custom messages that will keep them placated.

With the capsule implant, we have not only developed the capability to monitor an individual's medical state by tracking their behavior, we can easily determine if a person is happy or depressed, if they are having a heart attack or just having sex, or if they are getting exercise or are a couch potato along with a host of other metrics."

"That is fine from a medical perspective," Mel countered, "but what you are doing is monetizing all this data — data that is highly personal and private. And that is wrong."

"So you say," Alex said. "In our capitalistic culture, it is that monetization, as you call it that supports the systems and allows us to offer our medical services at a low cost."

"And what of the FDA regulations that say it is illegal to use implants like yours on healthy people?" Mel asked. "How is it possible for you to get around these regulations?"

"We made a case with government and the courts that all people are basically unhealthy in some way or another either now or in the future. Besides, the government was willing to set aside any ethical or moral issues to gain control of the people and reduce medical costs."

"So what you are doing is surveillance, pure and simple, in the guise of providing health care."

Their walk and talk had come to an end. They were standing in front of Alex's private elevator when a humanoid robot approached and handed Alex a sealed Petri dish containing one of the implant capsules. "And this is for you, little lady," Alex said.

Mel turned to run, but the goons were on her in a second and forced her into the elevator.

Arriving back in Alex's office, she was pushed face down and restrained on a gurney that had been placed there in their absence.

At the head of the gurney was a robot with a menacing gun-like attachment.

Alex handed the Petri dish to the robot who loaded the capsule into a chamber like loading a rifle. With one swift motion, the robot pressed it against the back of Mel's head at the base of her brain and inserted the implant painlessly with a sound no louder than that from the short puff of air from a compressor or a BB gun.

Alex said, "Resistance is futile. You are now mine."

With that, the thugs drove her home where she was shoved out of the slowly moving van onto the sidewalk in front of her apartment building. A bit skinned up and dazed, she realized, "These bastards know where I live."

CHAPTER SIXTEEN

As soon as Mel regained her composure after the shock of being abused by Alex, she realized that she had to have the implant removed immediately before the capsule became enmeshed in the growing tissue of nerves. A few doctors and other medical professionals were underground freedom fighters that she knew from protest meetings and social media. Among them was Dr. Bennett.

Arriving at the doctor's office, an assistant directed her to the examination room and told her to lie face down on the exam table.

Mel was still shaking as she told the doctor what had happened.

"Don't worry," the doctor said, "I see the small incision made by the applicator. It's neat and clean, about a quarter of an inch long. I'm going to inject you with a mild local anesthetic at the wound site, then open it up and extract the capsule with a small forceps so as not to damage it."

A few minutes later, Mel was sitting up and the doctor had the implant capsule in his hand. "Please have a seat in the waiting room for a few minutes while we prepare your implant clone," Dr. Bennett said.

Several minutes later, the assistant led Mel into a small office and gave her a thumb drive sized device in the form of a key fob. The assistant explained, "This device mimics your implanted capsule by sending fake health and location data back to Gordon. It will appear to their system as if you still had the implant in your body. Also, unlike the real implant which is powered by your body chemistry, this device needs a small battery that you will have to replace regularly."

Leaving the doctor's office, she felt woozy from the anesthetic. Her neck hurt and she had a headache. On the way to her car, Mel thought she saw some government goons watching her, but maybe she was just being paranoid because of all the abuse.

Driving home, she was so looking forward to a warm bath and a glass of wine followed by some much-needed sleep.

CHAPTER SEVENTEEN

Angelina, Alex's humanoid robotic assistant, ushered Sam Wagner, the party chairman, and Senator Frank Benson into Alex's spacious office. With handshakes all around, Alex welcomed the men and invited them to take a seat in one of the seating areas made up of four plush leather couches arranged around a large coffee table.

"Can I offer you some coffee or perhaps something stronger?" Alex asked.

Looking to Sam and replying for both men, Frank said, "Coffee will be fine, thanks."

"Now what can I do for you? Another big donation I suppose."

"No, you have been very generous in supporting the party," Frank said, "but we are here to make you a proposal. Through your leadership and the success of your personalized medication program, we have seen federal expenditures for drug costs reduced by ten percent. Some achieved because of the inability of other pharmaceutical companies to compete."

"Yes," Alex said, "I've been following the trends and I know that many companies have dropped out of the market which is pushing us into a near-monopolistic situation for some drug formulations."

Angelina returned and set a tray of coffee cups, a pot of hot coffee, and all the fixings on the coffee table.

Alex continued, "Don't get me wrong. I'm not the least bit worried about political or any regulatory push-back if we become a monopoly, which I doubt will happen because of all the other drug companies both foreign and domestic. So, what is your proposal?"

"We would like to make two proposals," Frank said. "First, since your medical implant capsule has become so successful, we are considering legislation to make the implants mandatory for people using the government drug program."

"Secondly," Sam interjected, "we would like you to consider running for president in the next election."

Everyone was silent as Alex considered the two proposals and what they would mean to his company's bottom line, not to mention his personal fortune. After taking a sip of coffee Alex said, "I'm flattered by your proposals and believe that mandatory implants will do a great deal to reduce the cost of our medical entitlement program, but I'm concerned that being president will cause me to divest myself of this company because of conflicts of interest regulations."

Frank spoke up and said, "Don't worry about that. Several of us in the Senate and House have discussed this. We think we can change the laws or at least drag any litigation through the courts using a variety of delaying tactics until your term in office has expired, at which point any legal argument will become moot."

"You don't have to decide now," Sam said, "but we are late in the election cycle and we need to launch your campaign soon so you can secure enough delegates leading up to the next convention."

CHAPTER EIGHTEEN

The business of performing the minor implant surgery was booming for doctors who were rewarded both by Gordon, who supplied the implants, along with the fees charged to the patients. The demand for implants also spawned a corresponding demand for implant clones. The government had made the clones illegal and was fighting to abolish them.

It troubled Mel to read reports that three doctors had died recently under mysterious circumstances and that the offices of Doctor Roger Bennett had been firebombed. Coincidently, all these doctors were those she had recommended to remorseful implantees who wanted to have their implants removed. Of course, Mel thought, there was no mention of them performing this surreptitious service in the news article.

Something was amiss, Mel suspected. This could hardly be a coincidence, she thought, but she didn't have a way to prove otherwise. Besides, what could she do? She had made recommendations to many implantees and could not remember who she talked to much less what doctors she referred them to. Clearly, she thought, there were those who were acting as spies and relayed her recommendations back to Gordon. In the interest of not placing doctors in danger, Mel stopped making referrals. If implantees wanted to have their implants removed, they would just have to find willing doctors on their own through word of mouth or on social media.

Doctor Bennett was a friend and someone who had taken part in several rallies. She felt somehow responsible for what happened, so she drove to his home to check in on him. Doctor Bennett's wife Elaine answered the door. Mel introduced herself and explained that she saw the news about the firebombing and was inquiring about the doctor.

Elaine, obviously very upset, lashed out at Mel, "I know who you are, and this is all your fault. If he hadn't gotten involved with you and your ridiculous privacy rights campaign... Elaine trailed off with her rant and Mel said, "I heard that there were injuries but no fatalities in the firebombing. I just stopped by see how Roger was doing and to find out if there was anything I could do."

"Roger was burned badly and is in the University Hospital," Elaine said, "and what you can do is to stop your foolish campaign and leave Roger alone. The issue is larger than all of us."

Mel thanked Elaine for the information and again offered to help, but Elaine slammed the door in her face.

* * *

A short time later Mel arrived at University Hospital. After a bit of persuading with the nursing staff in the burn unit, she was given a few minutes to talk with Roger.

Roger was bandaged almost head to toe and hooked up to oxygen, various beeping monitors, and several bags of dripping intravenous tubes.

At Roger's bedside, Mel asked, "How are you doing?"

"So far so good. I think I'll survive," he replied.

"I want to apologize if there was anything I did to put you into this situation," Mel said.

Roger held up a bandaged hand and said, "That's not necessary. I did what I did out of my own volition."

"Do you know who did this to you?"

Roger explained in a halting voice, "Not really. A few weeks ago, I was visited by some thugs in my office... and later in the parking lot who made some veiled threats... if I didn't stop removing the implants... but people were very troubled by what the implants were doing to them... and they needed help. All I know is that the police are looking into the matter. Now if you don't mind... I really need to rest."

Mel left the room as Roger faded off into a drug-induced sleep.

CHAPTER NINETEEN

Mel attended the party's political convention in Chicago. Like all such gatherings, it was a media circus complete with all the speeches, glad-handing, and schmoozing all taking place in an auditorium decorated with balloons, signs, and patriotic bunting.

Outside the venue, various protest groups came and went under the watchful eyes of police decked out in full riot gear who herded the people around like cowboys herding cattle to keep them in their stalls. Among these were a group of local Ban-The-Cap digital privacy advocates loudly trying to get the attention of the delegates.

Mel lent her support by rallying the demonstrators. She then used her press credentials to get a press pass that allowed her into the conference hall where she could interview many of the delegates. Employed as a stringer, a news service contracted her to write an article about the convention, so the thrust of her questions had to be about the politics of the moment. Among those questions were ones to solicit the thoughts of the delegates about the demonstrations. Most delegates were too wrapped up in the hype and celebrity of the events on the convention floor to be concerned about the demonstrators or their positions. When asked specifically about the Ban-The-Cap digital privacy issue, most of the delegates were aware of what they saw as the medical-related benefits but just shrugged off the privacy aspects saying that it was a small price to pay.

The highlight of the convention was the nomination of Alex Gordon to be the party's choice to run for election to the office of President of the United States. In his acceptance speech, Alex made a point of promising that, "If elected, my first action will be to improve health care for all and to reduce medical costs overall both for the individual and the government." He omitted how he would accomplish it and did not he refer to the medical implant capsule.

This had been a recurring theme or talking point throughout the campaign since Alex had announced his candidacy and the Ban-The-Cap protesters had made their presence known at all of his stump speech venues, and rallies over the past 9 months, much to his annoyance.

One of the conference events was an opportunity for the press to meet the candidate. When Mel tried to get Alex's attention to ask a question, Alex looked straight into her eyes. There was a recognition that he knew who she was, but he didn't acknowledge her raised hand.

CHAPTER TWENTY

When Mel returned from Chicago, she went straight to her apartment but found the street blocked by many police and fire department vehicles.

Pushing through the crowd of lookie-loos being held back by police, she told the nearest officer, "That's my apartment. I need to get through. Who's in charge here?"

The officer pointed to a man in a suit standing in the street, "Lieutenant Miller," the officer said.

Mel walked up to the Lieutenant just as someone in a body bag was being loaded into an ambulance.

Approaching the officer, Mel asked, "Lieutenant Miller?"

After she got the officer's attention, she said, "I'm Melinda Matthews and this is my apartment. What is going on and who is in the body bag?"

Looking up at the smoke still pouring out of the apartment's broken second-floor bay window, the officer explained, "About an hour ago, the fire department answered a call reporting a fire at this location. The building is not safe to enter, so we have yet to start our investigation. We have one fatality but no identification yet."

"When do you expect to know more, Lieutenant?"

"Give us a few hours. How about you meet me this afternoon at 3 at the 23rd Precinct Station?"

Mel thanked the Lieutenant and then went across the street where Bill and Deb Lewis, the first-floor tenants, were standing.

After a few minutes commiserating, Mel asked, "Did you by any chance notice or hear anything strange?"

"No," Bill said. "We had gone to the fitness center for our usual exercise class, then we did some grocery shopping. When we got back home, we saw smoke coming from your apartment and called 911."

"What are you going to do now?" Mel asked.

Deb replied, "I guess we will go to our son's place for a while. After we can get what's left of our belongings out of the apartment, we will have to find another place to live. How about you?"

"I have no relatives and no place to go. My only option is to get a cheap motel room somewhere."

Mel got back into her car and drove the short distance to Dave's Café where she sat nursing a coffee at a back table with her laptop computer. She still had almost four hours before her appointment with Lieutenant Miller. In a way, she felt fortunate that all her work had not been lost in the fire; it was all backed up in the cloud. She also had the clothes she took on the Chicago trip. There was not much in the apartment she cared about. Even old family photos and vacation pictures were on her computer and could be reprinted, but she felt bad for the Lewis family.

CHAPTER TWENTY-ONE

At 3 PM Mel went into the 23rd Precinct Police Station. Lieutenant Miller met her in the lobby and escorted her to an interview room where they were joined by another officer introduced to her as Detective Mattox.

"Have you been able to find out anything about the fire?" Mel asked.

"The investigation is ongoing, but so far it appears that the cause was a gas leak. We still don't have the ignition source," the Lieutenant replied," but we have to ask you a few questions."

"Am I under suspicion?"

"No, this is just routine. First," the Lieutenant continued, "can you account for your whereabouts yesterday and earlier today?"

"I've been in Chicago covering the convention for the past three days and just got back home early this morning. I was on my way home when I saw you on the street in front of my apartment." Mel rummaged in her purse, took out her airline ticket receipts, and slid them across the table to the officers.

Miller and Mattox looked at the receipts, then looked at each other. Without saying a word they gave the papers back to Mel.

"Does anyone live in the apartment with you?" Detective Mattox asked.

"No, I live alone."

Lieutenant Miller slid a photograph across the table. After a pause he asked, "Do you recognize this person?"

Mel looked at the picture. She knew the officers were observing her closely looking for her reaction or any tell, but she was still shocked and taken aback by what she saw.

"That's my brother, Jason," she finally said.

"Was he in the body bag I saw being taken away this morning?"

"I'm afraid so," Lieutenant Miller said. "I'm sorry for your loss."

"Don't be," Mel replied. "We've been estranged since we were teens."

"When was the last time you saw your brother?" Detective Mattox asked.

Mel told the officers about seeing him at the demonstration and later at her apartment. "But that was at least six months ago," she added, "and I haven't seen him since. How did he die?"

Opening a folder and flipping through a few pages, Detective Mattox said, "The medical examiner's preliminary report indicates that he died of smoke inhalation, but there were indications of blunt force trauma to the back of the head, so it's likely he was unconscious at the time of the fire. He was found lying on the floor in your apartment's living room."

"We would like you to go down to the morgue to make a positive ID," Lieutenant Miller said.

"I don't think so," Mel replied. "You can get his family, if he has one, to do that. Am I free to go?"

"Yes, you are free to go. Thanks for coming in."

CHAPTER TWENTY-TWO

Mel found a cheap motel on the outskirts of town. Her room had the odor of stale cigarettes combined with leftover sex. The abused furnishings and threadbare bedclothes were typical for a place that rented rooms by the hour, but she had no intention of being here long.

Opening her laptop, she saw an email with no subject line but tagged as important. This was typical of emails she usually disregarded as spam, but she was just plain weary from the travel, the fire, and the police interrogation, so in a moment of weakness she opened it anyway.

The message said "HAD ENOUGH?" in big bold letters. It was signed AG.

Slamming her laptop shut, she said, "That bastard!"

Sitting back on the bed, she thought, I guess so. I've had enough. Time for a change. But how was she going to extricate herself from all that she had started — all of her followers and a cause she believed in, which now seemed doomed?

She dozed off and was awakened several hours later by the rhythmic pounding on the thin wall coming from the next room. In her brief troubled sleep, she had an epiphany. She knew now what she would do.

Opening her laptop, Mel composed an email to her closest friends explaining what happened: the fire, the police, and all the gory details. She expressed how much she regarded their friendship, but that this would be her last email. She sent a similar email to her loyal helper, Tasha, and gave her all the administrative login information for the Ban-The-Cap social media and website. She wished Tasha good luck if she chose to carry on in her absence.

Finally, Mel deleted her email account. It was all so liberating. Now she could move on.

CHAPTER TWENTY-THREE

With the election of Alex Gordon to the presidency, Mel realized that despite all the efforts and dangers she and her like-minded followers put forth for more than a year, trying to warn the people of the privacy implications of the medical capsule implant seemed to mean little. She further came to understand that this was a big part of the raging issue on health care that had been front and center for several election cycles. This election confirmed that the people will willfully submit to surveillance, along with mind-control at the hands of big business, politicians, and the oligarchical elite. It was a valiant try, and Mel was comfortable with her decision to call it quits for now. Maybe

Elaine Bennett was right. The issue is larger than all of us.

* * *

At the Café de Paris overlooking the Mediterranean, Mel sat at an outside table enjoying her morning coffee. She reflected on what she had been through, thankful to be far away from the seemingly ever-present goons and musing about what to do next.

Roused from her reverie, Mel looked up to see a man standing next to her table. He appeared clean-shaven and well dressed in a casual sort of way.

"Mel?" the man asked.

Recognizing his voice, Mel asked, "Damon, is that you?"

"In the flesh," Damon replied.

"I didn't recognize you."

"New country, new me."

Mel gestured for Damon to have a seat and motioned to the waiter who came over to take his order.

"I wasn't sure you would see my text or if you would even meet with me," Mel said. "You may have sent a reply text, but I keep my burner cell turned off most of the time and generally live off the grid in a small village north of here these days to avoid being tracked. I assume you've heard what happened?"

"Yes, democracy, freedom, and individual privacy took a huge hit," Damon said. "At least here in Europe, the General Data Protection Regulation will keep the wolves at bay for a while, but I fear that even that will not be enough to keep the oligarchs from sucking up every individual on the planet into collective hives that they can manipulate."

Damon looked down into his coffee, then out at the Mediterranean. "It's so beautiful and peaceful here," he said. Then looking across the table at Mel asked, "So what are you going to do now?"

"I still do freelance writing for publications both in the U.S. and Europe under a pseudonym. I'm also working on a book about my experience as an activist that I hope will get some traction."

"Do you plan to go back?"

"I don't know. For now, I'm just lying low, enjoying the life of an expat, and reviving my high school French."

"Did you ever hear anything more from that whistleblower Wilson guy?"

"No, never heard from him again, but there is a good chance that he became carp food at the bottom of the river."

They both sat there a while longer in an awkward silence, savoring their coffees and feeling the fresh breeze blowing in from the Mediterranean. Making a promise to get together again, a promise neither of them had any intention

of keeping, they got up and went their separate

ways.

Acknowledgments

Thanks to our good friends Laura and Tim Shelley for being beta readers and for their helpful comments and edits.

* * *

Thank you for reading *The Implant.*

The website for this book can be found at www.TheImplantBook.wordpress.com where you are welcome to leave any comments and reviews.

Other works by this author can be found at:

www.flbob42.wordpress.com

www.RobertIveyStories.wordpress.com

www.vrbob.wordpress.com

www.ingramcontent.com/pod-product-compliance
Lightning Source LLC
Chambersburg PA
CBHW052147070326
40689CB00050B/2434